ACE Group Fitness Specialty Book

Traditional Aerobics

by Kathryn Bricker

CAUSEWAY
22 O'Meara St.
Ottawa, Ontario
K1Y 4N6

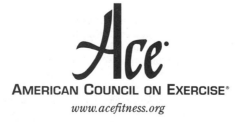

AMERICAN COUNCIL ON EXERCISE®
www.acefitness.org

Library of Congress Catalog Card Number: 00-106386

First edition
ISBN 1-890720-08-9
Copyright © 2000 American Council on Exercise® (ACE®)
Printed in the United States of America.

A B C D E F

Distributed by:
American Council on Exercise
P. O. Box 910449
San Diego, CA 92191-0449
(858) 535-8227
(858) 535-1778 (FAX)
www.acefitness.org

Managing Editor: Daniel Green
Design: Karen McGuire
Production: Glenn Valentine
Manager of Publications: Christine J. Ekeroth
Associate Editor: Joy Keller
Index: Bonny McLaughlin
Model: Jennifer MacBain

Acknowledgments:
Thanks to the entire American Council on Exercise staff for their support and guidance through the process of creating this manual.

NOTICE
The fitness industry is ever-changing. As new research and clinical experience broaden our knowledge, changes in programming and standards are required. The authors and the publisher of this work have checked with sources believed to be reliable in their efforts to provide information that is complete and generally in accord with the standards accepted at the time of publication. However, in view of the possibility of human error or changes in industry standards, neither the authors nor the publisher nor any other party who has been involved in the preparation or publication of this work warrants that the information contained herein is in every respect accurate or complete, and they are not responsible for any errors or omissions or the results obtained from the use of such information. Readers are encouraged to confirm the information contained herein with other sources.

REVIEWERS

Jeanne Blocher is the president of Body & Soul Ministries, an international, non-profit fitness organization that offers group fitness classes set to contemporary Christian music. Blocher is certified by Ken Cooper's Institute for Aerobics Research, as well as the American Council on Exercise, where she serves as an ACE Faculty member and practical trainer. She has been the choreographer and program designer for Body & Soul since it opened in 1981.

Ross Goo is a member of the American Council on Exercise's professional development department. In 1998, he launched a practical training system for new group fitness instructors, preparing them for the classroom setting. Goo has also been teaching traditional aerobics, step training, group indoor cycling, kickboxing, hip-hop aerobics, boot camp, circuit classes, and powerwalking for more than five years.

TABLE OF
CONTENTS

INTRODUCTION

The American Council on Exercise (ACE) is pleased to include Traditional Aerobics as a Group Fitness Specialty Book. Even as the industry continues to expand, evolve, and redefine itself, traditional aerobics remains a viable component of fitness. Guidelines and criteria have been established so that this exercise modality can be practiced both safely and effectively. The intent of this book is to educate and give guidance to fitness professionals that wish to teach traditional aerobics. As with all areas of fitness, education is a continual process. ACE recognizes this is a broad subject requiring serious study and we encourage you to use the References and Suggested Reading to further your knowledge.

Chapter One

Introduction to Traditional Aerobics

F ollowing the publication of Dr. Kenneth Cooper's book *Aerobics* in 1968, movement forms reflecting a shared cultural value of health and fitness proliferated. Traditional aerobics was among these, tracing its early lineage to such pioneers as Jacki Sorensen, founder of Aerobic Dancing, Inc., and Judi Sheppard Missett, president of Jazzercise, Inc. These women and others adapted Dr. Cooper's concept of aerobic exercise to exercise classes with music, creating what became known as aerobic dance-exercise or, simply, aerobics. With the release of "Jane Fonda's Workout" video in 1982, the dissemination of traditional aerobics to a mass market via electronic media forever changed fitness culture worldwide. A 1986 survey published by the International Health, Racquet, and Sportsclub Association (IHRSA) showed that 21.9 million people in the United States participated in aerobics that year. The gender bias of the activity was noted by International Dance-Exercise Association (now IDEA, the International Association of Fitness Professionals), which reported in 1986 that 93.8% of its members were female.

American Council on Exercise statistics showed this trend to be holding, reporting in 1999 that 94% of ACE-certified group fitness instructors were female.

Growth

Though statistical data show a downtrend in general participation in the 1990s (American Sports Data, Inc., 1996), traditional aerobics continues to provide the form, methodology, and objectives upon which subsequent group fitness forms have been modeled. When combined with step aerobics, American Sports Data statistics show participation in 1996 in the United States alone to be 34 million. A 1997 IDEA programming survey reported that of the three primary types of traditional aerobics (high-impact, combination high-low impact, low-impact), only high-impact aerobics was on the decline. Both low-impact and mixed-impact aerobics appeared stable with 85% and 73% of survey respondents, respectively, offering these classes on their weekly schedules. It is noteworthy that the percentage of clubs offering low-impact aerobics was surpassed only by step aerobics at 86%. Class sizes in general are reported to be smaller, though the diversification and specialization of class types no doubt accounts for some of this.

Benefits

A primary benefit of traditional aerobics is the social interaction and sense of community that develops from frequent participation and promotes adherence and motivation. In addition to these psychological and motivational benefits, aerobics also provides many of the benefits of physical fitness: aerobic endurance, muscular endurance, muscular strength, flexibility, and improved body composition.

Kinesiology

The potential for freedom of movement is greater in traditional aerobics than many other traditional modes of aerobic training. Only the anatomical limits of the body and the boundaries of the room dictate the form of the movement. By selecting movements that foster biomechanical balance, you can prepare participants for the movement challenges of daily living. Biomechanical balance is achieved when the flexibility and strength of all muscles surrounding a joint are adequately balanced (Figure 1). You can create this balance in two ways: 1) select movements that balance one another within the context

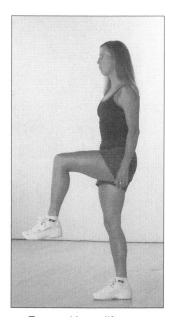

a. Forward knee lift

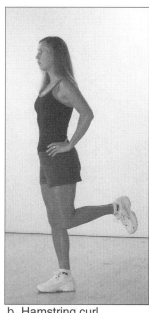

b. Hamstring curl

Figure 1
Select movements that achieve biomechanical balance.

of the class and 2) select movements that correct the imbalances created during daily movement patterns.

Movements that balance one another within a class session should be evaluated in four ways:

1) Is there a balance between the major muscle groups and joint actions? For example, chest presses can be balanced by scapular adduction.

2) Is there a balance in the quantity of movements performed? For example, 16 repetitions of biceps curls can be balanced by the same number of triceps extensions.

3) Is there a balance of spatial paths? For example, forward movements can be balanced by backward movements, and movements in the sagittal plane can be balanced by movements in the frontal plane.

Figure 1
continued

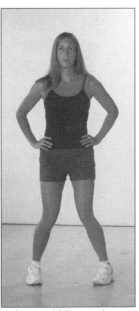 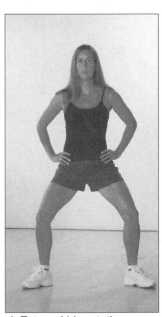

c. Internal hip rotation   d. External hip rotation

4) Are both halves of the body used equally? For example, lead arm/leg patterns can be regularly alternated between right and left.

To correct the imbalances created during daily movement patterns, observe for habitual postures, and then design movements that restore neutral, symmetrical, and functional alignment. This usually involves stretching and strengthening muscles, and giving instructions to foster improved alignment. For example, suggest that participants pull in their abdominals to encourage activation of the transversus abdominus for improved pelvic alignment. Ellison (1996) recommends counterbalancing "the slouched, round-shouldered, flexed-leg positions of the professional sitter" by emphasizing "spinal extension, scapular retraction, hip and knee extension, and dorsiflexion."

Chapter Two

Choreography

Musical Interpretation

T
he basis of musical interpretation lies in understanding the relationship between the rhythmic patterns of movement and music. A common denominator in the rhythmic experiences of both movement and music is their temporal organization, in that they share the characteristics of time, such as duration, pulse, and pace. Although rhythmic structures are based on much more, their time patterns provide a starting point for elementary studies in synchronizing music and movement. The benefit of using music in classes is that it provides an underlying structure, systematically progresses the movement, makes upcoming movement changes predictable, and evokes feelings and expression.

Moving to the Beat

No other instructional deficiency is likely to result in as swift or thorough a rejection by class participants as the inability to move to the musical beat. Similarly, participants who cannot move to the beat disrupt and distract others. Therefore, you must not only be skilled at moving to the beat, but also in teaching this skill to others.

Beats are defined as regular pulsations that create an even rhythm, much like the steady ticking of a clock. Individual beats are of equal duration. A series of beats forms the underlying rhythm that synchronizes the music and the mover. Poor room acoustics or hearing impairment can result in participants being unable to hear the musical beat. Inability to move to the beat can also result from exaggerated states of neuromuscular tension. When a mover is too tense, encourage him or her to relax, embody the beat, and be moved from within. Because the breath provides a fundamental organizing rhythm in the body, have participants vocalize on each beat to coordinate exhalations with movement exertions. Hand clapping to the beat is both a movement and a sound, and can enhance rhythmic awareness by simultaneously providing kinesthetic, auditory, and tactile experiences.

Musical beats alternate stressed and unstressed pulses. The stronger pulsations are called **downbeats**, while the weaker pulsations are called **upbeats**. The sense of the upbeat is critical to developing a mover's sense of timing. The movement preparation often occurs on the upbeat so that the exertion is timed on the downbeat. Since faulty preparation leads to faulty execution, simple drills for developing the sense of the upbeat are encouraged. These can be as simple as marching to the downbeats while clapping the upbeats or repeating four skips (hop-steps) on counts "and-1-and-2-and-3-and-4" followed by four walks on counts "5-6-7-8."

Determining the Tempo

The **tempo** is the rate of speed of the steady pulsation, expressed as beats per minute (bpm). Because music tempo directly affects movement intensity, selecting appropriate tempos for various class segments and populations is of primary concern. Furthermore, if tempo/range-of-motion compatibility is compromised by excessive speed, participants are unable to execute movements safely. This can be observed when weight remains on the balls of the feet during running because the music is so fast that the heels do not have time to lower. Select tempos that accommodate the largest movements, and then adapt smaller movements to that tempo. For example, long lever arm circles with sideward traveling footwork will require more time to execute with proper form and control than stationary marches with biceps curls. If the tempo is set to accommodate the first movement, the marches can be adapted by raising the knees higher, or lowering and raising the center of gravity. Observe participants carefully and adjust tempos accordingly. Taller people with longer limbs cannot perform the same movements as quickly as people with shorter limbs. Other factors such as age, time of

There is no one correct system for counting music. The difference between "dancers' counts" and "musicians' counts" has long been noted in musicians preferring to count "common time" in groups of four (1-2-3-4) and dancers preferring to count in groups of eight (1-2-3-4-5-6-7-8). Dancer's preferences for feeling the larger groupings has also been noted in certain meters of music by their counting just the strong pulsations while musicians count both strong and weak. Among musicians, various preferences for counting have been observed depending on musical style and meter. Because the basic sense of proportion in time is not affected by the system of counting, the underlying musical structure remains intact. Fitness instructors, therefore, should expect and tolerate differences as they adapt from various systems in their own application.

day, familiarity with the movements, and individual body structure can all influence how the tempo affects individual movers.

Identifying the Meter

The **meter** of a song organizes the underlying pulse into groups of beats having a primary stress on the first beat of the group. Each group of beats is referred to as a measure or bar of music. To identify the meter, listen for the regular occurrence of a strong accent in the steady pulse. Count each strong accent as "one" and the subsequent beats as "two-three" and so forth until the next strong accent. The number of beats counted before the next strong accent is the number of beats per measure. It is this aspect of metrical organization that is most relevant, as it provides the foundation for the structure of the movement. All musical meters are based upon multiples or combinations of two fundamental meters known as **duple meter** and **triple meter**. Duple meter is groupings of two beats ("boom-chick") and triple meter is groupings of three beats ("boom-chick-chick"). The first beat of each measure receives primary emphasis. Most music used in classes is written in 4/4 meter, also known as "common time," which is a duple-based meter, as four is a multiple of two. The first four indicates that there are four beats to a measure of music. The second four indicates that the quarter note receives the beat.

4/4   4 beats to the measure; accent on 1st beat; quarter note gets the beat.

An example of a triple-based meter is 6/8, in which the six indicates there are six beats to a measure. The eight tells us that an eighth note receives the beat.

6/8   6 beats to the measure; accent on 1st beat; eighth note gets the beat.

Though less common, utilizing triple-based meters in certain class segments can create rhythmic variety that is refreshing to participants. Motivation and adherence can suffer from the monotony of classes feeling like one endless march. Gavin (1997) points out that moving in "novel ways" changes neural patterning as the brain "adapts to new stimuli." He adds that participants can experience this as both "liberating" and "risky." Utilizing the affinities that exist between musical meter and spatial shapes can foster both biomechanical and psychological movement balance. According to Tech (1994), the "difference between a 3/4 and a 4/4 is that the 3/4 has a moment to breathe. So a 3/4 is a rounder, fuller, softer, swinging motion; it is circular. A 4/4 is not circular; it is square. It has greater strength and drive; it gives more energy to the body."

Recognizing the Phrases

A **phrase** in music is like a sentence in written or spoken language. As letters of the alphabet combine to form words, and words combine to form sentences, so beats of music combine to form measures, and measures combine to form phrases. To learn to recognize musical phrases, imagine where you would pause for a breath if you were singing a song. A musical phrase must be composed of at least two measures of music and can be of any length. It has become standard in fitness classes to work with 32-count phrases that are counted as four groups of eight counts each. To track the groups of eight counts in a phrase, you can count "1-2-3-4-5-6-7-8, 2-2-3-4-5-6-7-8, 3-2-3-4-5-6-7-8, 4-2-3-4-5-6-7-8." If notating the phrasing, a slash can indicate each eight-count phrase, with a slash across the group for the last count of each phrase. For example, one 32-count phrase would be written as ⊔⊔⊔⊔ ⊔⊔⊔⊔ ⊔⊔⊔⊔ ⊔⊔⊔⊔. When working with music that is not produced for 32-count phrasing, analyze the song by notating it in this manner. If a regular pattern establishes itself, movements can be structured to synchronize. If, however, there is irregular phrasing or the phrase does not end in an even measure, techniques for dealing with musical "glitches" can be employed, such as extending the repetitions of a preceding movement or performing 2-count movements, such as kicks, until the regular musical phrasing reestablishes itself.

Feeling the Rhythm

There is a difference between **rhythm** and rhythmic patterns. Any sound or movement has a rhythm, but when it is established and repeated it becomes a pattern. When rhythm is defined as a regular pattern of movement or sound that can be felt, seen, or heard, what is actually being referred to is a rhythmic pattern. Because movement and music have time in common, aerobics choreography primarily focuses on blending the time patterns of musical and movement rhythms. One popular method of choreography emphasizes creating secondary rhythms in movement to overlay consistent and predictable musical phrasing. The rhythms of aerobics movement are generally designed to synchronize with the music rather than interpret it. Musical interpretation results more from matching musical and movement styles such as, for example, in funk or hip-hop aerobics. Movement patterns lay secondary rhythms over 32-count blocks of music primarily by altering the duration of movements and placing accents. For example, the duration of movements can be varied by executing at half-tempo (two beats per movement), regular tempo (one beat per movement), or double-time (one beat per two movements). For example, accents can be added in one of three ways when walking: by moving with greater force, such as stamping one beat; by moving with greater range, such as stepping out further; or by moving with greater dynamics, such as clapping certain beats.

Syncopation is defined as shifting the accents that fall on the normally stressed beats in the underlying rhythm to unstressed beats or parts of beats. Mettler (1979) points out that "any beat, except the first beat of the measure, can be syncopated. The weaker the beat, the more syncopated it becomes when it is emphasized. The second half of a divided beat can provide a particularly strong feeling of syncopation." An example of syncopation is to hold (no movement) on count 1, run right-left on count "and-2," walk right on count 3, and walk left on count 4. The emphasis on count "and 2" is created by moving with greater force and range.

Selecting Appropriate Music

The majority of instructors purchase tapes and CDs that are produced specifically for aerobics classes. Among the features these tapes offer are even phrasing, formatting for class components, appropriate style, and licensing. Most selections have a driving beat that motivates participants. Occasionally, instructors prefer non-metered music as a backdrop for individually timed movements synchronized with the breath. Experiment with different styles of music to avoid monotony and determine participants' preferences. Seasonal music for holidays and specialty tapes for theme classes can add festivity and fun. Aerobic music services offer a wide variety of musical styles, class formats, and tempo ranges, making it easy to select appropriate music. For instructors who have the equipment and resources, compiling original music for classes is an option.

Typical bpm ranges for class components:
>   Warm-up: 120–140 bpm
>   Low-impact aerobics: 120–140 bpm
>   Combo hi/lo-impact aerobics: 130–170 bpm
>   High-impact aerobics: 150–170 bpm
>   Aerobic cool-down: 120–130 bpm
>   Muscular conditioning: 110–130 bpm
>   Flexibility training: <100 bpm

Movement Patterning

The language of movement has its own grammar and syntax. As movement unfolds in space and time, an underlying kinesthetic logic binds its flow. The craft of the choreographer is to pattern the flow of energy that creates movement. The term **choreography** literally means the designing or writing of circles, and is used by fitness instructors to denote the planning and composition of structural movement.

Types of Choreography

Francis (1993) identified two types of aerobics choreography, the **structured method** and the **freestyle method**. She defines the structured method as "movements that are formally arranged and repeated in a predetermined order (and) usually performed to the same piece of music each time the routine is used." Judi Sheppard Missett's Jazzercise and Jacki Sorensen's Aerobic Dance are cited as examples. An advantage to using the structured method is the ability it gives the choreographer to interpret musical passages with specific expressive movements. This can be very satisfying to the participant. Structured choreography also allows the participant to master movements and know what is coming next. For some individuals this predictability can create a "comfort zone." A disadvantage of this method is the lack of flexibility it provides for adjusting the progression of movement based on participant response.

Francis defines the freestyle method as using "movements that are built and sequenced by the instructor during the aerobics class." The obvious advantage to the freestyle method is the ability to adjust the movement progression as it unfolds. For example, a specific movement could be repeated more or less depending on how quickly the participants master it. Decisions on how to progress the complexity, intensity, or impact of movements can be made as you observe the class.

Inherent to the success of the freestyle approach is the ability to adjust movements to the musical phrase. For example, if a footwork pattern is repeated until the majority of participants are performing it successfully, you must be able to sense the upcoming musical phrase in order to correctly time the introduction of the next development in the sequence. Until this skill is fully automatic, perform drills outside of class time to master it. Constructing drills from one's own choreography can provide specific rehearsal. For example, a drill could be developed by sequencing two basic movements, each with one variation.

Basic Movement Variations

Basic Movement #1:	Grapevine (step side, cross-back, side, tap; counts 1–4)
Variation #1:	Replace tap on count 4 with ball-change on count "and-4." (This creates a temporal variation in the rhythm commonly called a rhythmic variation.)

By altering the number of repetitions for each part of the sequence and practicing it to different musical selections, you can develop the skill for responding spontaneously to musical phrasing.

The skill of adjusting to the musical phrase is dependent on mastery of two more elementary skills, the first of which is structuring movement that synchronizes with the musical meter. Since most music used in classes is 4/4 meter, which has four beats to a measure, it is necessary to structure movement patterns based on the equivalent or multiples of four. For example, if a grapevine based on 6 counts (step side, cross-back, side, cross-front, side, tap) were performed alternating to the right and to the left using 4/4 meter music, one would soon sense being out of synchronization with the musical phrase. Restructuring the step to be based on 4, 8, 16, or 32 counts (e.g., reducing the 6-count grapevine to 4 counts [side, cross-back, side, tap] or by expanding it to 8 counts by adding two marches counts 7 and 8) could eliminate this problem.

It is necessary to know what numerical beat corresponds to what movement in order to initiate count 1 of the movement pattern on count 1 of the music. For example, knee lifts could be performed with a step on count 1 and a knee lift on count 2 or a knee lift on count 1 and a step on count 2. Lack of clarity as to where the sequence begins and ends, as well as what movement is performed on what count, results in movement patterns that are neither predictable or repeatable, or synchronized with the musical phrasing.

According to Francis (1993), "Freestyle movements can be sequenced either by using **linear progressions** or by placing movements into patterns or **combinations**. A linear progression consists of one movement that transitions into another without cycling sequences. . . . Combinations are defined as two or more movement patterns combined and repeated in a sequence several times in a row." The obvious advantage to using linear progressions is that participants do not have to remember what came before. For example, you could lead the class in step-touches for 16 counts, then add arm work for 16 counts; the arm work could be maintained as the leg work is changed to hamstring curls for 16 counts; the leg work can be maintained as new arm work is introduced for 16 counts and so forth. No movements in the sequence are repeated. Using linear progressions simplifies the learning process for beginners by allowing them to respond to cues and self-monitor intensity levels. Because linear progressions feel less choreographed, they may be more appropriate for teaching participants who prefer routines that are not too "dancey." Often, instructors employ linear progressions in a segment of a class that is otherwise based on combination building. This most frequently occurs in the warm-up or when introducing new movements. The advantage to using linear progressions when introducing new movements is that you can focus on teaching proper technique, such as how to execute a pivot safely. The movements introduced as linear progressions might be included later in a combination.

In combination building, begin with the simplest kinetic idea, usually a basic movement, then add, subtract, or change one element at a time until the final pattern or combination is formed. Changing only one element at a time increases the likelihood that the participants will follow the movement progression successfully and maintain an appropriate heart rate. Combinations are then linked sequentially (A+B+C).

Movement Classification

Movements using the feet as the base of support are classified as being either axial or locomotor. **Axial movements** occur above a stationary base where the body can rotate around its own axis but holds a fixed spatial point. The central axis of the body does not travel through space (e.g., squats and turns). **Locomotor movements** are movements in which the central axis of the body changes its location as it travels through space (e.g., extended runs and slides).

There are four fundamental locomotor movements upon which all others are based. A **walk** is defined as a step in which weight is transferred from foot to foot with one foot always remaining in contact with the ground. The weight during a walk typically sequences from heel to toe. A **run** is defined as a step where there is a momentary loss of contact with the ground as the weight shifts from foot to foot. The weight during a run typically sequences from forefoot to heel. In a **hop**, the body weight is propelled off of the ground from one foot with the landing occurring on the same foot. In a **jump**, the body weight is propelled from one or both feet with the landing occurring on both feet. These four fundamental locomotor movements are based on even rhythms. Each component of the movement is executed with the same time value when performed naturally. For example, as the mover walks, he or she would naturally perform each step to a steady cadence.

Three other movements, the **skip**, **slide**, and **gallop**, are combinations of the four basic locomotor movements and are based on uneven rhythms, in which one component of the movement is performed to a greater or lesser time value than the other component. This creates an uneven subdivision of the beat. In a skip, a step and a hop are performed sequentially on the same foot as the mover alternates feet. In a slide, the mover steps sideways then draws the other foot up to the first with a quick transfer of weight. In a gallop, the heel leads the step forward followed by a quick close of the other foot to it. As the weight shifts onto the second foot, the knee of the first leg is raised. The skip, slide, and gallop are of a higher complexity level than the four basic locomotor movements.

The weightbearing leg in any movement is called the **working leg**. When one leg is not bearing weight, such as in a knee lift, the non-weightbearing leg is called the **gesturing leg**. For example, in standing hamstring curls the step on count 1 is performed by the working leg and the hamstring curl on count 2 by the gesturing leg. Being able to distinguish the action of the working and gesturing legs aids in analyzing and breaking down movement. Most basic movements used as the starting point when building combinations are based on variations and combinations of axial, locomotor, and gesture movements. For example, a "step-touch" is a step (work) to the side on count 1 and a tap (gesture) of the other foot on count 2. An example of a neutral movement is a jumping jack, in which both feet jump apart on count 1 and together on count 2.

Elements of Variation

Basic movements can be varied by altering their space, time, and force characteristics. Although the space, time, and force elements of movement are organically inseparable (changing one will affect the others), for the sake of analysis, we divide them (Figure 2).

> Space is about "where."
> Time is about "when."
> Force is about "how."
> Body is about "who/what."

The expression **elements of variation** was coined by Copeland (1987) to describe ways in which base moves could be altered. Copeland's five elements of variation (lever, planar, directional, rhythmic, and intensity) provide a base from which other creative instructors continue to expand. Spatial elements of variation are those that have to do with where the movement occurs.

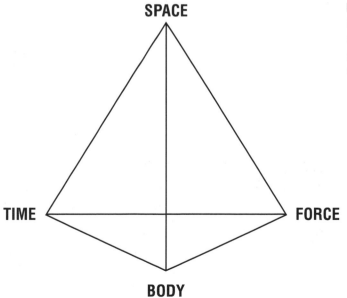

Figure 2
Model of choreographic elements of variation

For example, a planar variation is created by changing the path of the movement from one plane to another (e.g., changing forward kicks [sagittal plane] to side kicks [frontal plane]). A directional variation is created by altering the path of movement that the central axis of the body follows as it travels across the floor (e.g., stationary kicks can be traveled forward, backward, sideways, diagonally, or circularly). The spatial range or volume of a movement can be varied by increasing or decreasing the size of arm circles or pendulum leg swings. Spatial range is also adjusted by lever variations when, for example, a long lever arm or leg is changed to a short lever. The level of a movement (center of gravity relative to floor) can be varied, such as when walking high on tiptoe, then low in a crouch. A particularly rich source of choreographic variety can be found in spatial variations of group formations. For example, divided along adjacent walls, group A performs a stationary movement as group B travels, then group

Figure 3
Spatial variations in group formations. Group A performs a stationary movement as Group B travels.

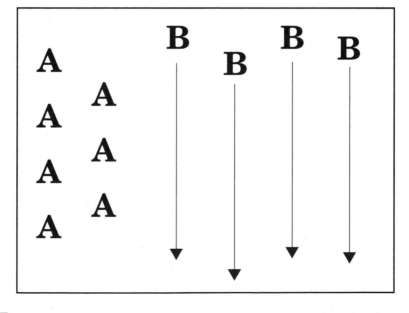

B performs a stationary movement as group A travels and so forth (Figure 3).

Temporal elements of variation change "when" the movement occurs. The most commonly used are rhythmic variations, which alter a movement's rhythm to create more or less movement per unit of time. For example, seven walks forward at regular tempo on counts 1-7 with a tap on count 8 could be changed to two half-tempo walks on counts 1-2, 3-4, three regular tempo walks on counts 5-6-7 with a tap on count 8, thereby creating less movement per unit of time. To create more movement, the rhythm could be changed to eight double-time walks on counts "and-1-and-2-and-3-and-4," three regular tempo walks on counts 5-6-7, and a tap on count 8. Other examples of temporal variations can be seen when successive movements are employed, such as when timing successive arm movements in a group of exercisers to create a "wave" or a "centipede." Instructors manipulate the temporal elements of movement to create different feeling tones in the movement. Laban (1974) describes this as changing the mover's "attitude towards time" along a dimension from "quick" to "sustained." Without changing the quantity of time in which a gesture is executed, it could be performed with an eagerness to arrive at the destination (quick) or a lingering quality in which focus on the point of departure predominates (sustained). For example, a leg gesture could be performed with the eagerness of stomping on a spider or the reluctance of dipping a foot into a cold lake.

Manipulating the force factors in a movement changes how it looks and feels both quantitatively and qualitatively. Movements can be performed with a sense of strength and increasing pressure or with a sense of lightness and decreasing pressure. Gavin

(1997) emphasizes the psychological impact of this element of variation by noting "strong movements convey a sense of assertion and control. . . . When you choreograph with strong movements, you enable participants to access their power and feel in charge. . . . Light movements. . . are important choreographic elements because they foster a sense of delicacy and sensitivity (and) can help participants connect with an inner state that corresponds to effortless movement."

These elements of variation are by no means all-inclusive. It is in the manipulation and combination of these elements of variation that the excitement and vitality of movement comes alive.

Transitions

A class that flows smoothly from one movement to the next is the result of effective **transitions**. Transitions connect individual movements to one another, and blocks of movement to other blocks. Knowing where movement A ends, where movement B begins, and what movements are needed to connect A and B are the keys to building effective transitions. Three primary factors influence how well one movement transitions into the next. The first is the position of the body or body part(s) in space. The ending position of movement A must correspond to the beginning position of movement B or a connecting movement must be created. For example, if both arms press overhead, sideward, downward, and forward on counts 1–8, the ending position for movement A is hands next to the body with elbows flexed. If movement B is triceps kickbacks, the transition from movement A to B will be smooth. If, however, movement B begins in a different position than movement A ends, such as with long-lever lateral arm raises, movements to bridge A and B will be needed.

The second factor to consider when building transitions is the direction of the movement. If the direction of movement A differs from B, the movements should be sequenced so as to avoid potential injuries from awkward changes of direction. An example of effectively transitioning a change of direction is seen in warm-ups when movement A is forward-facing step taps (feet wide) and movement B is sideward facing rear ankle extension/flexion (feet stride). To transition from A to B, movement A is gradually turned sideward.

The third factor affecting transitions is weight distribution. For example, if movement A is a grapevine (step right, cross-back left, step right, tap left; counts 1–4), the ending position is weight distributed over the right leg. For a smooth transition, movement B could begin with a transfer of weight to the left leg, a propulsion (hop or jump) off the right leg, or a gesture of the left leg.

A particular class of transitions that creates lead leg reverses is important for maintaining biomechanical balance. To reverse the lead leg, a movement must either end in a neutral stance (weight over both feet) or result from an uneven number of weight transferences. Examples of movements ending in a neutral stance are variations of jumps and knee bends such as jumping jacks, scoots, and squats.

Three techniques are commonly used for creating an uneven number of weight transferences using 4/4 meter music. The first is to replace one count with a non-weight-transferring movement. This could be accomplished by walking on counts 1-2-3 and tapping or clapping on count 4. A second technique is to subdivide a musical beat with a "quick-quick" weight transfer such as by walking on counts 1-2-3 and "run-running" on count "and-4." A third technique is to perform a "single-single-double" pattern of a movement such as lunges or knee lifts.

Another special class of transitions is performed when you are switching from mirroring the class to facing the same direction. To be effective these transitions must not only be correctly performed but also clearly cued, such as by saying, "You hold here. I'm going to turn to join you." If explicit directions are not given the class can become confused and mimic you as you switch directions. Some of the techniques for transitioning to "mirror image" are similar to those used in lead leg reverses with the addition of a half-turn. For example, performing a half-turn on a neutral move (or substituting one for an existing step) can be effective. Substituting a "single-single-double" pattern with a half-turn on the double as the class performs four single repetitions of the same movement can also be effective. For example, as the class performs four alternating knee lifts, perform two alternating knee lifts then a double knee lift as you half-turn. Another effective transition is to substitute a weightbearing movement with a half-turn for a gesture movement. For example, in step taps, the tap on count 8 could be replaced by another step with a half-turn.

Choreographic Building Techniques

There are four primary techniques for building movement patterns. Their purpose is to progress the movement sequence in a manner that allows participants to follow easily while maintaining appropriate heart rates. The first choreographic building technique is **repetition reduction**, or pyramid building. In repetition reduction, the number of times each movement in a sequence is repeated is gradually reduced until the final pattern is achieved. For example, four different 2-count movements, such as jumping jacks, forward heel taps, backward lunges, and knee lifts, could be repeated eight times each, then four times each, then two times each.

The second choreographic building technique, **rhythmic variation**, has several applications. As discussed earlier, rhythmic variations alter a movement's rhythm to create more or less movement per unit of time. New movements can be introduced at half-tempo so that they are learned at a slower pace. This strategy is particularly effective for teaching movement sequences that do not break down well. Because heart rates drop if movement is slowed down for too long, sequencing half-tempo movement introductions in the warm-up or at the beginning of the aerobic component can be more effective. Rhythmic variations also are used to progress the complexity or intensity of movements, such as when movements are performed double-time to the musical beat.

The third building technique, **add-on**, is especially effective for teaching longer movement sequences. One movement is taught, and then the next movement is added. Both movements are then repeated before the next movement is added. For example, movement A could be taught for 16 counts, then movement B could be taught for 16 counts to create a 32-count block of movement. Movements A and B could then be repeated for 8 counts each and movement C added for 16 counts to complete the 32-count block. Movements A, B, and C could then be repeated for 8 counts each and movement D added for 8 counts.

The skill of adjusting movements to the musical phrase is critical to success in applying this technique.

The fourth building technique is **layering**, in which options for changing intensity, complexity, and impact are superimposed on established movements. For example, a grapevine alternating right then left could be established; arm work could be added to increase both complexity and intensity; the center of gravity could be raised and lowered, further increasing intensity; a hop could replace the tap on counts 4 and 8, increasing impact, intensity, and complexity; both feet could leave the floor on count 2, further increasing impact, intensity, and complexity. As each new option is layered over an existing movement, participants can choose whether to stay with the existing movement or progress to the next level. Once the options have been presented, continue to demonstrate the various levels rather than always progressing to the highest level, particularly when teaching newer participants.

Chapter Three

Teaching a Traditional Aerobics Class

Verbal Introduction

Begin each class by introducing yourself and identifying newcomers. Inform participants of the level and type of class, as well as the sequence and length of class components, and any risk factors associated with the workout. For example, participants who leave early should be cautioned to perform their own aerobic cool-down. Pain felt in or around a joint during a particular movement should be regarded as a sign to discontinue or modify. A technique review could include items such as how to pivot properly or execute a new movement, as well as methods used for monitoring intensity. For example, go over cues for pulse counting, to improve accuracy and demonstrate recommended modifications, such as how to modify impact or intensity.

Equipment

Equipment needed for aerobics classes includes:

Sound system with variable speed tape deck and/or CD player

Wireless microphone, rechargeable batteries, and battery recharger

Resilient, non-skid floor surface

Clock or watch with second hand

Heart rate and rating of perceived exertion (RPE) charts

Mirrors (optional)

Instructor platform (optional)

Resistance apparatus such as hand weights, elastic tubing, and stability balls

Mats for floorwork

Supportive shoes

Footwear

Because foot structures vary, no one shoe is appropriate for everyone. Provide educational handouts on shoe selection to assist participants who ask for recommendations. According to Rizzo (1999), "Foot experts report that a poor shoe-to-activity match is frequently a factor in sports-related lower extremity injuries. . . . The biomechanics of aerobics involves substantial lateral movement and quick, multi-directional changes. Impact focus is on the ball of the foot."

A well-chosen aerobics shoe, which should be replaced every 100 hours of use, has the following features:

- Firm sole, yet flexible forefoot
- Well-cushioned midsole

- Sturdy upper with comprehensive lacing system to stabilize the foot
- Roomy toe box
- Lightweight construction
- Mid-cut design for additional heel support
- High-top design (for those with ankle problems)

Cueing

The purpose of cueing is to prepare participants for upcoming movements or give feedback, instruction, motivation, or correction. Effective cueing promotes exercise safety by ensuring participants move in synchronization with the group, transition smoothly into new movements, and perform movements correctly. The two types of cues are verbal and visual. Verbal cues require knowledge of safe and effective use of the vocal apparatus. Visual cues are hand signals or movement demonstrations that provide information. Both types of cues give information about who, what, when, where, why, and how. For example, "who" could refer to beginners in a multilevel

Figure 4
A sampling of Oliva's
visual cues for exercise
classes based on the
principal of visual-gestural
communication and
American Sign Language.
(Source: Oliva, 1988)

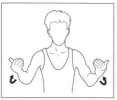
"MOVE IT FORWARD"
(travel toward me)

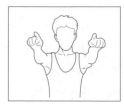
"MOVE IT BACK"
(travel backwards)

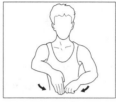
"STEP TOUCH"*

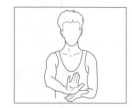
"HEEL DIGS"*

These four visual cues are foot movements;

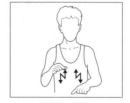
"MARCH IN PLACE"

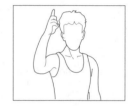
"ONE MORE"
(repeat the step/sequence
one last time)

class; "what" could refer to a body part or an action; "when" refers to timing; "where" refers to space; "why" states purpose; and "how" instructs.

Oliva (1988) developed a standardized visual cueing system that utilizes hand signals (Figure 4). The benefits of this system are that it can reach large groups, protect the voice, accommodate the hearing-impaired, and counter poor room acoustics. A second set of visual cues, the Aerobic Q-signs, was developed by Webb in 1989. Both cueing systems are currently used by group fitness instructors. Another type of visual cueing is **visual previews**, in which participants continue performing established

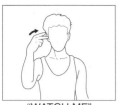

"WATCH ME"
(new move: watch and
copy; – ASL: Look at me)

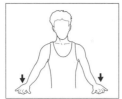

"STAY IN PLACE"
(stop traveling – ASL: Stay)

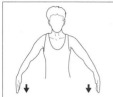

"TOE TOUCH"*

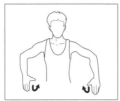

"LIFT THE HEELS"*

notice your hands approximate what your feet do.)

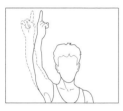

"SINGLES"
(as opposed to "doubles"
or "repeaters")

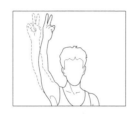

"DOUBLES"
(do a movement twice with
the same arm and leg)

Verbal Cueing

Griffith (1982) identifies the following common types of verbal cues:

Footwork cues – tell "what" foot to use

Directional cues – indicate "where" to move, such as forward or backward

Rhythmic cues – indicate "how" to time a movement relative to other movements, such as slow (2 counts) or quick (1 count)

Numerical cues – count "when" an action occurs rhythmically, such as counting "1-and-2-3-4" to describe the rhythm of "kick, ball-change, walk, walk"

Step cues – name "what" the action shall be, such as a jumping-jack movements while you demonstrate a new movement. Body language corrections for proper alignment and form are another type of visual cue. For example, raise then lower the shoulders to demonstrate correct positioning.

Determining the order of information and correctly timing cues are important instructional skills. The most effective ordering of information depends upon context. For example, if transitioning into a new movement, counting down "8-7-6-5," then naming the action "grapevine," and direction "right," followed by "go" with two double-time claps (motivational cue) can provide an effective strategy. The order of information for the next cue will again depend on context. If a modification is offered, identifying "those wanting to increase intensity," followed by demonstrating and saying "add a hop," can be effective. Timing of cues depends on context as well. When cueing a movement change, time cues well enough in advance of the change so that participants can accurately respond. For example, a new step beginning on count 1 of a phrase will need to be cued on counts 5 and 6 of the previous phrase. If the new movement falls on counts 5-6-7-8, as can happen when movements are layered over established movements, then the cue will come on counts 1 and 2. Although cues should be concise, the length of cues can vary, affecting how far in advance they should begin. For example, with beginners, a countdown from the beginning of the preceding phrase, "8-7-6-5," then "grapevine right" on the last 4 counts may prepare them more effectively than just cueing "grapevine right" on the last 4 counts. Alternately, when giving a visual preview, verbal cues are often given simultaneously to describe and reinforce the action. Numerical and rhythmic cues are typically delivered as the movement they describe is being performed.

Spatial cues refer to one of three orientations, or systems of reference (Guest, 1995). For example, when giving the directional cue, "arms forward," to what does the word "forward" refer? The first system utilizes body orientation; all movements are described in reference to body structure "without concern for outside points of reference." In the example, arms forward refers to in front of the body whether the exerciser is standing or lying supine. The second system places the body's central axis in relationship to the line of gravity, so up and down remain constant, but the mover's personal front can be carried into various directions. To continue the example, arms forward refers to the front of a vertically upright body, which could be facing various directions. The third system is based on geographic orientation, and movement is described in reference to the environment. One wall of a room is usually established as "front" and directions are given accordingly. In the example, "arms forward" refers to a constant environmental reference point, so the mover could be reaching behind his or her body toward a forward wall. As is obvious from the example, the spatial key and movement must be effectively matched for clarity. Unless circumstances dictate using another key, directional orientation is generally used. Geographic orientation, however, can be more effective when the same movement is repeated facing various directions. For example, "walk-2-3-tap" could be established traveling forward and backward, then quarter-turned each repetition to travel to front, side, back, and side walls (geographic orientation). In movements where the body axis is off-vertical from the gravitational pull, such as in push ups, or rotating around its own axis, such as in turns, cues using body orientation can be more effective. In addition to appropriately matching movements and spatial keys, words for cueing spatial orientation should be carefully selected. For example, when lying supine, cue to stretch a body part headward, footward, chestward, tailward, skyward, or earthward. Such terms, if appropriate, can be more specific and less confusing than, for example, cueing upward, downward, forward, and backward.

Injury Prevention

Early studies showed that the majority of injuries associated with high-impact aerobics resulted from overuse and occurred in the foot and lower leg (Garrick et al., 1986). As participants and instructors became more educated and low-impact techniques were developed, traditional aerobics became safer. To avoid overuse injuries, a gradual progression of exercise impact, intensity, frequency, and duration is essential. The rate of progression should be based on factors such as a person's health status, aerobic fitness level, age, and personal goals. The data needed for determining an appropriate rate of progression can be generated through pre-exercise screening. When this is combined with proper technique, floor surfaces, and shoes, an acceptable level of exercise safety can be achieved.

Technique

Even a safe exercise, if performed incorrectly, can result in injury. A knowledge of biomechanics enables you to observe participants for proper form, anticipate common errors, and provide effective correction techniques. Perform all movements with control and within a normal range of motion for the joint(s) involved. Be aware of, and avoid, the mechanisms for injury associated with each joint. Generally these include movements considered to be too repetitive, excessive, fast, or ballistic. Equally emphasize stability and mobility in movement. For example, when performing overhead arm work or leg movements involving hip flexion, emphasize stabilizing a neutral pelvis (Figure 5). Other areas of proper technique include rotating the palms to face upward when abducting the arms above shoulder level, limiting weightbearing knee flexion to 90 degrees, guiding the knees over the feet when bending, and decelerating impact forces by rolling through the foot.

Contraindicated/High-risk Movements

1. Hyperextension of joints

2. Excessive repetitions on weightbearing leg

3. Flinging limbs

4. Rapid change of direction

5. Prolonged amount of time on the balls of the feet

6. Extended holding of the arms at or above shoulder level

7. Unsupported lumbar spinal forward flexion

Environment

You are responsible for providing a safe exercise environment, which includes the following:

1. A resilient, dry floor surface that is clear of unmarked obstacles

2. Adequate floor space per participant

3. Appropriate ventilation and room temperature

4. Availability of water

5. Phone in case of emergency

6. First aid supplies

7. Safe music levels, including audible cues

8. Emergency evacuation plan

9. Charts for monitoring exercise intensity

10. Operational and safely stored equipment

Optional

11. Mirrors

12. Raised platform for instructor

Encourage participants to use sweat towels to avoid slipping on wet floors, keep liquids in non-breakable, covered containers, and wear supportive shoes.

Figure 5
a. Correct form for stabilizing a neutral pelvis during overhead arm movements.
b. Incorrect form

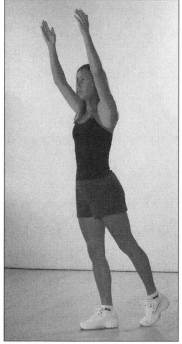
a.

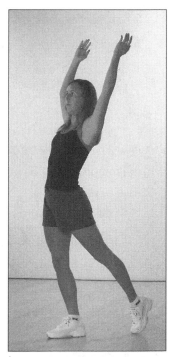
b.

Personal Limitations

Health

Be aware of medical disorders that affect exercise, as well as the health histories of participants. All participants should complete a health history screening prior to taking your class. You can then recommend specific modifications, as well as be prepared to respond to emergencies should they arise. Planning class activities with appropriate modifications for specific medical conditions is essential for providing all participants with a safe exercise session. For example, instruct participants who are taking beta blockers, which can affect heart rate, to monitor exercise intensity using rate of perceived exertion instead. Show

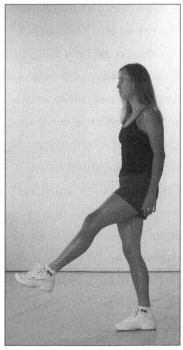 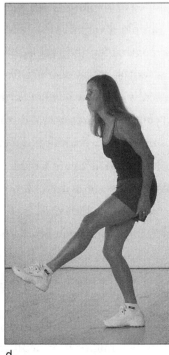

c. Correct form for stabilizing a neutral pelvis during a forward kick.
d. Incorrect form

c.

d.

pregnant exercisers beyond their first trimester alternatives for exercises in supine position. Instruct hypertensive exercisers to avoid sustained isometric contractions, such as when performing holds to increase intensity during abdominal curls. Make educational handouts available to exercisers with special conditions such as diabetes, arthritis, exercise-induced asthma, and pregnancy. Handle information regarding medical conditions with sensitivity and respect for a person's privacy.

Fitness

Measuring participants' major components of physical fitness enables you to recommend and monitor safe levels of exercise. Record results on file cards for review. In addition to increasing safety, this method can motivate participants by establishing short-term goals and tracking progress. The information acquired can guide participants when selecting appropriate modifications. For example, a very fit athlete may be weak in core body stabilizing strength. Identifying this through testing could help this person select the safest exercise from the suggested modifications. A person with a low level of cardiovascular fitness, for example, could control progression of duration by performing the remainder of the aerobic segment at a cool-down level after having sustained target heart rate for the appropriate amount of time. Similarly, a person with a high level of body fat or an inflexible foot structure, as indicated by high arches, could limit impact.

The information from fitness testing can also be used to identify muscle imbalances that, if left uncorrected, could lead to exercise injuries. For example, tight hip flexors are associated with excessive lumbar lordosis, which predisposes a person toward low back pain. Tight calf muscles limit range of motion at the ankle, which makes it difficult to adequately absorb impact.

Identifying and correcting potential problems can help to avoid many injuries.

Modifications

Modifications are movement options that allow individuals to adapt exercises to an appropriate level. The range of options you offer will vary with the type and level of the class, but, generally, classes require a multi-level teaching approach. Individuals differ in skills and fitness levels, as well as in specific fitness parameters, such as flexibility at a particular joint, so classes must be planned accordingly. When teaching healthy populations that have been properly screened, most modifications for aerobic training are designed to adjust the movement intensity, complexity, or impact. More fit and skilled individuals can adapt group movements to be appropriately challenging, yet safe, by selecting from the modifications offered. The choreographic building technique, layering, is particularly effective for generating options within an aerobics sequence. It is important to provide a visual model of the various modifications and not remain just at one level. Additionally, as special populations mainstream into regular classes, you will need to be familiar with participants' health histories so that more specific modifications can be offered.

Modifying for Intensity

Movement intensity is based upon "how much body mass must be moved how far in what amount of time" (Clippinger, 1993). Because the center of weight and the greatest mass exist in the lower body, modifications involving the lower body will normally have the greatest impact on intensity. Incorporating intensity-monitoring techniques and eliciting feedback will ensure that individuals make appropriate choices in modifications designed to adjust intensity (Figure 6a).

How much body mass is moved can be affected by the number of body parts involved and lever length. Studies in bench stepping, in which movement ranges and tempos were controlled, have demonstrated that exercise intensity increases by adding arm work (Francis & Francis, 1992). Layering arm patterns over established footwork is a viable means of adjusting intensity (Figure 6b). Over-reliance on overhead arm movements to increase intensity is discouraged, however, due to studies indicat-

Figure 6a
Basic grapevine; step side on count 1, cross-back on count 2, step side on count 3, return to starting position on count 4

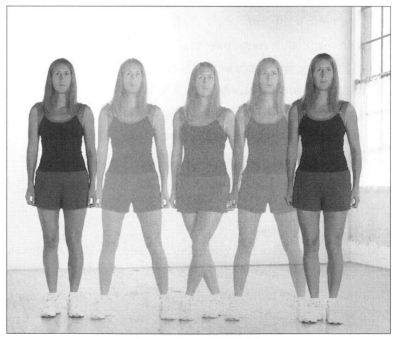

ing this technique creates heart-rate responses that are dispro-
portionately high for the oxygen consumption normally associated with them. This can be misleading and result in under-train-
ing. Another technique for increasing how much body mass is
moved is lifting a limb or body segment. For example, a lateral
leg lift could be layered over count 2 of a step tap. A third technique, lever length modifications, can also modify intensity (e.g.,
layering straight leg kicks [long lever] over knee lifts [short lever]).
Studies indicate that the risk/benefit ratio of adding hand or ankle
weights to augment body mass precludes their use for peak cardiovascular training in aerobics classes (Francis & Francis, 1988).

Figure 6b
Adding armwork; arms out to the side on count 1,
overhead on count 2, out to side on count 3, back
to starting position on count 4

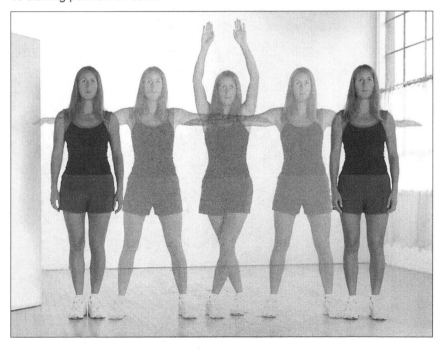

How far the body mass is moved can be affected by any modification that changes a movement's range. For example, intensity can be increased by raising the knees higher, lowering and raising the center of gravity, traveling more, or adding hops and jumps (Figures 6c & d). Participants can be observed to automatically modify the range of movements. You should determine whether this is occurring because of the individual's habitual movement patterning or in response to music tempos and movement intensities.

Raising and lowering the center of gravity is another effective modification to increase intensity. The center of gravity in an up-

Figure 6c
Raising and lowering the center of gravity;
knees and hips flex on counts 1 and 3, and
extend on counts 2 and 4

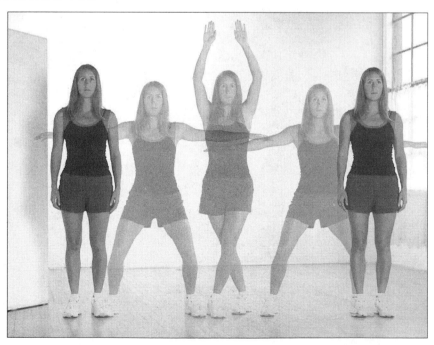

right stationary body lies approximately in front of the second sacral vertebra, allowing variance for build and alignment. For example, establish side taps without level change for participants needing lower-intensity modifications, and then superimpose increased flexion of the knee and hip to create a level change. You can also increase intensity by adding propulsions, which propel the center of gravity into the vertical dimension.

A fourth technique, traveling more, increases the range in which the center of weight moves in the horizontal dimension. Studies in both step and traditional aerobics have demonstrated that adding traveling to choreography significantly increases

Figure 6d
To change a movement's range, propel from the floor on count 2. Another option is to add a side leg lift, ball-change, or hop on count 4.

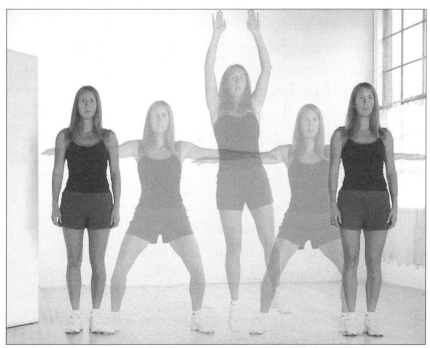

movement intensity. Otto (1988) showed that emphasizing traveling in low-impact aerobics can create oxygen and metabolic costs comparable to those generated by high-impact aerobics.

Since all participants are moving to the same tempo music, intensity modifications that manipulate the amount of time in which the body moves must be created by layering rhythmic variations over the steady beat. For example, walks at regular tempo could be established as a lower-intensity modification, then skips to a subdivided beat can be superimposed as a higher-intensity modification.

Modifying for Complexity

Complexity is based upon the amount and type of information that must be processed per unit of time. A gradual progression of complexity with well-planned breaking down and building of movements is critical for participant success. Know the types of movements associated with various skill levels and observe for errors and give appropriate feedback. Adjust the movement progression according to participant response, as less-skilled individuals will become frustrated with movements that are too complex, while more experienced participants will become bored if not sufficiently challenged. When instructing multi-level classes, emphasize movement variety vs. complexity to keep the majority of participants motivated and successful.

The types of movements associated with different skill levels can be understood within the context of the developmental movement patterns from which they emerged. The human infant develops through stage-specific movement patterns that continue to inform the more complex patterns of adult movement. By revisiting these earlier patterns, you can modify movement complexity. In one of the earlier stages of development, the central axis of the body forms, creating spinal movements. Moving the spine along its vertical dimension, such as when lowering and raising the center of gravity through knee bending, provides low-level movement complexity. As movements progress to the next stage, the upper- and lower-body differentiate in bilateral patterning, in which both arms and/or legs perform the same action (e.g., jumping jacks). In the next stage, the body differentiates its right and left sides, and homo or ipsilateral movements appear in which limbs on the same side of the body move together. The final stage of development brings contra-lateral patterning, in which limbs on the opposite side of the body move together. You can modify complexity by moving in either direction along this developmental path. For example, a progression could sequence spinal (knee bends), bilateral (both arms abducting), then unilateral movements, which could be either ipsi-lateral (taps right/left, adding same-side arm abducting) or contra-lateral (taps right/left, adding opposite arm abducting).

Each individual also has a personal history in which certain movements are familiar and others are not. Because "the temporal and spatial features of the motor program are based on past experience," previous experience should also be considered when selecting movements (Simmons, 1998). For example, participants familiar with footwork patterns to music from other movement forms generally adapt to aerobics choreography more readily than participants who have none. New movements that are similar to those taught in class the previous week will seem less complex than new movements that are dissimilar to any done before.

You can control the amount of information offered per unit of time by changing how you build movements and the number of body parts involved. For example, movement sequences can be condensed to varying degrees by repetition reduction. A 16-count phrase with four knee lifts (8 counts) and four tap sides (8 counts) is less complex than condensing to an 8-count phrase with two knee lifts (4 counts) and two tap sides (4 counts). Changing only the footwork is less complex than footwork and arm patterns combined. Additionally, certain variations of movements are inherently complex, such as turns and quick transfers of weight as seen in "ball-changes." Present these variations as advanced modifications by layering them over existing movements. Participants can then opt to remain with the simpler versions if the complexity of the advanced modification is too challenging.

Modifying for Impact

Be prepared to present all movements with well-planned modifications for impact. Despite a class being listed as high-, combination-, or low-impact, participants of varying levels often attend because the time is convenient. In facilities that offer fewer classes on their schedules, all levels may be combined into one class by necessity. Success in applying this instructional skill requires knowing both high- and low-impact versions for all movements, as well as being able to demonstrate these options by layering them over established movements. Attending other instructors' classes and observing professional videos will help you develop inventories of the most effective modifications for standard movement vocabulary. Often, adaptations are as simple as altering the distance the feet travel from the floor. For example, marches, prances, or runs can be used interchangeably to provide respectively low-, moderate-, or high-impact options. A second technique for modifying impact is to add or delete hops and jumps. For example, hamstring curls can be performed step right count 1, curl left count 2 (low-impact), or step right count 1, curl left and hop right count 2 (high-impact). A third technique is to substitute one step for another, such as taps side (low-impact) for jumping jacks (high-impact). Steps that are substituted for one another should be based upon the same number of beats, as well as begin and end similarly so as to transition smoothly into other movements.

The major class types in traditional aerobics — low-, moderate-, and high-impact — are based upon modification of impact. Impacts are defined as a collision between the feet and the floor. Two types of impact are created when a foot contacts the floor: 1) **vertical impact**, which exerts forces upward through the foot, and 2) **horizontal impact**, in which friction makes the foot slide less easily across the floor. Studies have shown that for specific movements, such as a step-tap, vertical impact forces are greater when the step is performed high-impact, while horizontal impact forces are greater when the step is performed low-impact (Francis & Francis, 1989). When experiencing vertical impact, the foot and lower leg are more vulnerable; with horizontal impact the knee is more vulnerable. By controlling and varying impact forces, as well as matching the appropriate type with the participants, a greater degree of exercise safety can be maintained.

Low-impact Aerobics

During low-impact aerobics, one foot remains in contact with the floor at all times. Intensity is varied by range of motion, amount of muscle mass, lowering and raising the center of gravity, tempo, and traveling. Beginner, deconditioned, obese, senior, and pregnant exercisers generally require low-impact aerobics. Most individuals can benefit from this type of training as low-impact does not mean low-intensity. Low-impact is not suitable for people who need to avoid prolonged knee flexion, are excessive pronators, or cannot achieve sufficient overload for cardiovascular benefits. The vertical impact forces associated with low-impact aerobics are 1 to $1^1/4$ times body weight (Francis & Francis, 1989, *High- and low-impact aerobics*).

Moderate-impact Aerobics

During moderate-impact aerobics, one foot is kept on the floor at all times while the center of gravity is lifted then lowered by raising onto the ball of the foot. Rather than flexing the knee and lowering the center of gravity, movements are initiated by an extension of the knee and ankle as the center of gravity is raised. To experience the difference between low- and moderate-impact technique, move from a march to a prance. Moderate-impact technique gives the feeling of bounce without the abrupt impact associated with high-impact aerobics. Vertical impact forces associated with moderate-impact aerobics are 2 to $2^1/2$ times body weight (Francis & Francis, 1989, *Moderate-impact aerobics*).

High-impact Aerobics

During high-impact aerobics, both feet momentarily lose contact with the floor as the body is propelled into space. Running, jumping, leaping, and hopping movements are all high-impact. For conditioned individuals who remain injury-free, high-impact aerobics provides a challenging workout. A large muscle mass is required to propel the body from the ground, and then decelerate when landing. Because high-impact movements feel different from low-impact movements, certain individuals prefer one or the other based on qualitative differences. High-impact aerobics is generally not suitable for deconditioned, senior, obese, or pregnant exercisers, or for people who suffer from shin splints or incontinence. The vertical impact forces associated with high-impact aerobics are more than 3 times body weight (Francis & Francis, 1989, *High- and low-impact aerobics*).

Combination Hi/Lo-impact Aerobics

During "combo hi-lo" aerobics, movements are alternated using high- and low-impact techniques. The advantage of this approach is that it varies the type of impact and accommodates a broad range of participants. Because some participants will perform all movements low-impact, select movements that adapt well either way. Select music tempos that accommodate both high- and low-impact techniques. Additionally, movements must be sequenced to transition smoothly from high to low to avoid a choppy feeling, which certain combinations can give.

Chapter Four

Programming

Components

Class design progresses through warm-up, peak work, and cool-down phases. The specific components, sequence, and length vary depending on factors such as instructor/participant preference and class emphasis. For example, you may split up the muscle-conditioning segment by performing standing upper-body strengthening following warm-up and floor calisthenics for the remaining muscle groups after the aerobic cool-down. A 45-minute lunchtime class may emphasize aerobics and exclude muscle-conditioning altogether. The following sequence is intended as an example of a 60- to 75-minute class.

Warm-up

The purpose of a warm-up is to prepare the body for the more vigorous activity to follow. This can be accomplished by continuous rhythmic movement utilizing the large muscles of the body to elevate core body temperature, rehearse upcoming movements, and stimulate the cardiorespiratory and neuromuscular systems and metabolic energy pathways. The progression of intensity should be sufficient to elevate core temperature 1 to 2°F and raise heart rates toward the lower end of the training zone. Participants should begin to focus on listening for instructor cues, moving with others, and monitoring body sensations. Warm-ups in traditional aerobics generally last five to 10 minutes, but the amount of time needed will vary depending on class profile, time of day, and intensity, sequence, and type of workout.

The types of movements used in warm-up can be classified as general or specific. General movements are those that contribute to the preparatory phase of the workout, but do not rehearse upcoming movements. General movements elevate core temperature, enhance kinesthetic awareness, or provide specific muscle group/joint warm-up. For example, pliés raise core temperature, but need not be included later in the peak work of a high-impact class. Standing pelvic tilts teach neutral pelvic alignment while enhancing kinesthetic awareness. Toe taps and shoulder rolls can provide needed muscle group/joint warm-up.

Specific movements create a rehearsal effect by mimicking movements to be used in the workout, but at a slower pace and lower intensity. For example, linear progressions or simple combinations of upcoming aerobic movements raise the core temperature while they provide rehearsal. Other specific movements rehearse the mechanics of their more active counterparts, such as when performing push releases to practice jumping mechanics (Figure 7).

In sequencing warm-up movements, gradually progress intensity, range of motion, and complexity, while striving for biomechanical balance. As long as movement flows logically and supports the physiological, biomechanical, and psychological goals of the warm-up, there is no particular rule of order. Various approaches can be effective. For example, a gradual progression might favor placing smaller movements for body awareness such as head isolations, shoulder rolls, and pelvic tilts at the beginning, and then progressing into whole-body movements. When working with beginners who may have underdeveloped kinesthetic awareness, such exercises can provide needed movement education to enhance performance and safety. Another strategy for more advanced participants favors beginning with whole-body rhythmic movements and layering smaller, less active movements over them. Because there is so much to accomplish in 5–10 minutes, designing an effective warm-up is a challenging task.

Figure 7
Push releases

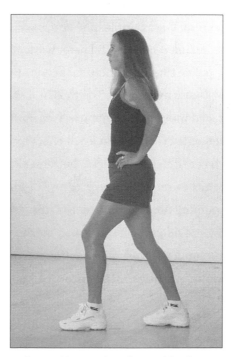

a. Start with your foot flat and body weight forward.

Use the following checklist when reviewing a warm-up:

1. Is there sufficient stimulus to all major muscle groups/joints?

2. Is this stimulus applied in a balanced way?

3. Do the selected movements provide sufficient rehearsal?

4. Is there a gradual progression in range of motion, intensity, and complexity?

5. Does the music tempo allow movements to be performed through a full range of motion with control?

6. Are the goals of the warm-up achieved?

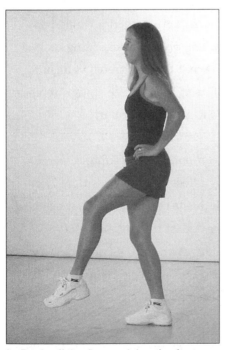

b. Push off the floor, raising the foot slightly.

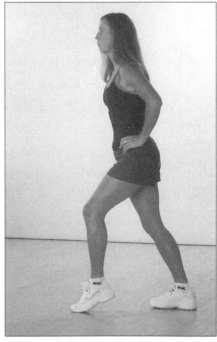

c. Land gently on the forefoot and roll back onto the heel.

Pre-performance Stretching

There is a consensus that stretching for muscle elongation is not appropriate during the preparatory phase of a workout. The role of pre-performance stretching, as distinguished from stretching for muscle elongation, is an area of debate. The goal of pre-performance stretching is the same as that of warm-up: to prepare the body for the upcoming activity. Utilizing dynamic stretches or progressively larger range-of-motion movements supports other preparatory goals such as elevating core temperature. On the other hand, static stretches in warm-up are rarely held longer than 10 to 12 seconds. If properly integrated with more active movements, this should not significantly reduce body temperature. For example, a calf stretch could be held briefly as the upper body remains active, then a whole-body active movement could follow. The question regarding its role in aerobic warm-up centers on what type of stretch to include (dynamic vs. static) and how, if used, to integrate static stretches in order to support the metabolic goals of warm up.

Aerobics

The purpose of the aerobic component is to enhance cardiovascular fitness and favorably affect body composition. The American College of Sports Medicine recommends that exercise intensity be 65–90% of maximal heart rate (MHR) or 50–85% of maximum heart rate reserve, duration of 20–60 minutes, and frequency a minimum of three days per week. Because the risk of muscloskeletal injury increases as intensity, duration, and frequency of training increase, gradual progression is essential. Most classes perform aerobics for 20–30 minutes saving longer sessions of 40–50 minutes for advanced participants only. When determining the duration and intensity of the aerobic component, the optimum risk-to-benefit ratio depends on many factors, including participant profile, class type, and objectives. For example, individuals whose goals are health-related will better comply to a moderate program that keeps them free of injuries. Elite athletes require challenges that are beyond the training goals of the average person. Deconditioned individuals will need to reduce the intensity and duration of aerobic training while the musculoskeletal system adapts.

Aerobic benefits are achieved by using either a continuous or intermittent format. The **continuous format,** also called steady-state training, is the more common method. Following the 5–10 minute warm-up, intensity is gradually increased until target heart rates are achieved. Target heart rates are sustained for the duration of the aerobic component, and then a 5–10 minute cool-down progressively lowers intensity to below training levels.

To sustain a steady-state heart rate, select movements to provide physiological balance. For example, if low-impact movements are combined with high-impact movements, elements of variation can be employed to maintain consistent exercise intensity. Perform low-impact marches while lowering and raising the center of gravity to maintain an intensity comparable to high-impact kicks. Perform smaller-range movements double-time to match the intensity of larger-range movements.

In **intermittent training**, or interval training, bouts of intense activity are alternated with recovery periods. The length and intensity of the intervals vary depending on the participant profile and class objectives. Often the higher-intensity interval crosses the anaerobic threshold with participants working at 85% of maximum heart rate or above. The active recovery interval is used to pay back the oxygen debt. For example, participants may perform 90-second anaerobic intervals with heart rates at 85–90% of MHR followed by three-minute recovery intervals with heart rates at 65–70% of MHR (Figure 8).

When teaching multi-level classes, it is important to select movements for the anaerobic intervals that beginners can modify. For example, establish step-tap side at the conclusion of the lower-intensity interval, and then layer leap-tap side over for the anaerobic interval. Give beginners the option of remaining steady-state by continuing to perform the lower-intensity version. One benefit of this interval design is that more energy can be expended in the same amount of time as a result of performing the higher-intensity work.

Another popular form of intermittent training alternates aerobic and muscle-conditioning intervals. The muscle-conditioning

Figure 8
Continuous and intermittent exercise

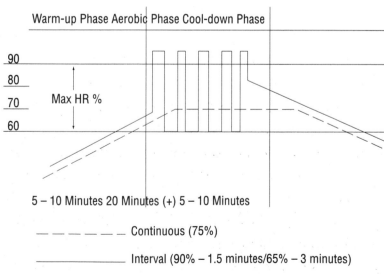

Warm-up Phase   Aerobic Phase   Cool-down Phase

90
80
70   Max HR %
60

5 – 10 Minutes   20 Minutes (+)   5 – 10 Minutes

– – – – – – Continuous (75%)

———————— Interval (90% – 1.5 minutes/65% – 3 minutes)

intervals are usually designed to sustain target heart rates by involving upper- and lower-body movements simultaneously. For example, alternate a four-minute aerobic segment with heart rates at 75–80% of MHR with a four-minute muscular-conditioning interval with heart rates at 60–65% of MHR. Participants enjoy this format because it offers variety and they can accomplish muscle conditioning and aerobics training at the same time.

Aerobic Cool-down

Following aerobics, perform 5–10 minutes of lower-intensity work to reduce heart rates to the lower end of the target zone. The objective is to prevent blood pooling, hasten removal of metabolic waste products, and reduce muscle soreness. Because cardiac complications are more prevalent with the cessation of exercise, performing a cool-down is critical for ensuring safety. The large muscles of the lower body should continue contracting isotonically to assist the pumping of blood from the lower body

---

Consider the following when designing intermittent training:

1. Determine the goals.

2. Determine the work/recovery ratio.
   (For example, a one-minute work interval followed by a three-minute recovery interval is a 1-to-3 work/recovery ratio.)

3. Determine the number of cycles (one work/recovery repetition) needed to create a set (the total number of cycles). (For example, a 30-minute segment could be composed of three sets of 10-minute cycles alternating five minutes of high-intensity aerobics with five minutes of lower-intensity muscle conditioning.)

4. Select appropriate movements to meet the goals.

back to the heart. A common error instructors make is having participants sustain isometric contraction in the lower body, such as with a held squat, when upper-body strength training is merged with cool-down. Continue to flex and extend the hips and knees to avoid blood pooling. Additionally, do not lower, then raise, the head below heart level as this can cause dizziness.

Muscular Conditioning

Muscular conditioning components, which generally last 15–20 minutes and utilize some form of external resistance, are designed to enhance muscular strength and/or muscular endurance. Traditional strength training isolates individual muscles groups and trains muscles for maximum force production. Traditional muscular-endurance training also isolates muscle groups, but uses lighter loads and higher repetitions. Functional strength training focuses on the whole body as an integrated unit and trains muscles in the roles they play in daily movement patterns. For example, the stabilizing role of the abdominals is emphasized along with the moving role in trunk flexion. When designing muscular conditioning components, decide which approach (traditional or functional) or combination of approaches best meets the class objectives. Exercises with appropriate modifications can then be designed to meet those goals.

Flexibility Training

The final class component, which generally lasts from 7 to 10 minutes, is stretching and relaxation. At this time conditions are optimal for achieving flexibility gains as tissue temperatures are high (Pollock & Wilmore, 1990). Because stress reduction is a primary reason people exercise and stretching promotes relaxation, this final class component can provide needed balance. Techniques such as breath awareness and stillness can promote a mindset conducive to stretching. Participants should relax the muscles prior to moving into the stretch. Pay particular attention to those muscle groups that, if tight, can predispose the exerciser to injury: the gastrocnemius-soleus complex, hip flexors, anterior shoulder, low back, and hamstrings (Figure 9a–f). Various stretch techniques can be incorporated, such as static and PNF stretching. Avoid rapid, high-force, or ballistic stretching. To accommodate varying levels of flexibility, select stretches that have a mechanism for adjusting intensity. For example, bending the knee during a hamstring stretch can reduce intensity. For beginners, incorporate stretches that isolate individual

Figure 9a
Gastrocnemius stretch

Figure 9b
Soleus stretch

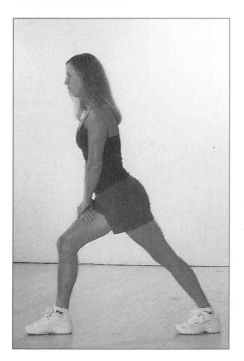

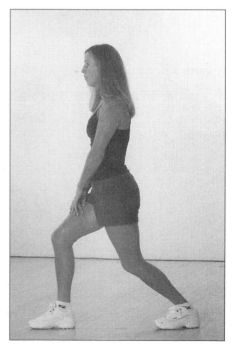

muscle groups and do not require balance. A thorough knowledge of joint biomechanics and stretching techniques is essential for safe and effective stretching.

Intensity Monitoring

Exercise intensity refers to the severity of the work being performed or the physiological overload. If exercise intensity is too low, a person will not receive cardiovascular benefits. If exercise intensity is too high, a person can be injured or unable to continue the exercise session. Monitoring exercise intensity helps ensure that each individual exercises at an appropriate level. The appropriate method or combination of methods will vary, depending on factors such as your expertise, available data, the exercise program, and the participant's health status, fitness level, and experience. The two practical

Figure 9c
Deep lunge stretch for the hip flexors

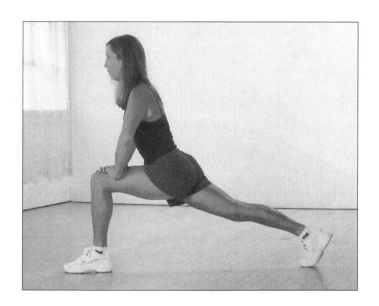

methods for measuring exercise intensity in an aerobics class are pulse monitoring and RPE.

During steady-state training, check intensity levels approximately 10 minutes into the aerobic component and then a second time before the aerobic cool-down. When intermittent aerobic training is employed, a subjective method, such as RPE, is often utilized to enhance class flow. Following aerobic cool-down, check heart rates to be sure they are at or below 120 bpm. If individuals are found to have a heart rate higher than this, they should keep the lower body moving until cool-down has been achieved. The class profile, format, and objectives will influence how and when exercise intensity is monitored. For example,

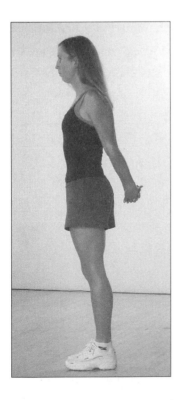

Figure 9d
Anterior
shoulder
stretch

Figure 9e
Supine stretch for
the low back

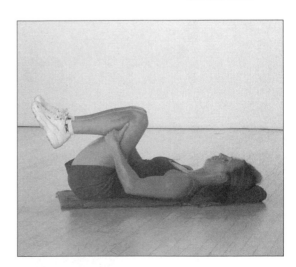

beginners can benefit from comparing RPE levels with heart rates to develop kinesthetic awareness and may need to monitor intensity more frequently. Experienced exercisers, however, may be very accurate in subjectively assessing intensity.

Variations

Programming variations can be based on differences in class objectives, formatting, or style. For example, sports-conditioning programs are designed to train athletes for the specific challenges of the activity. Drills that replicate the movement skills and energy systems associated with the sport are highlighted. Circuit classes are programming variations based on class formatting. The term "circuit" refers to a number of exercises arranged consecutively. In aerobic-circuit training, participants move from one station to the next, performing activities designed to improve cardiovascular conditioning. In

Figure 9f
Hamstring stretch

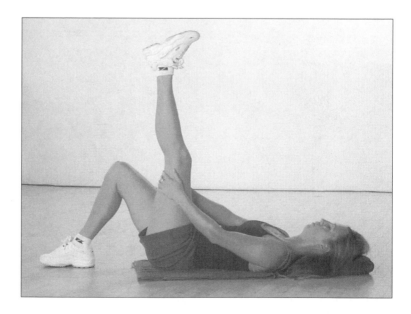

some formats, aerobic stations are alternated with muscular conditioning stations. Another common source of program variation is found in different styles of dance-based classes such as funk, hip-hop, Latin, African, ballet, folk, and modern dance-based fitness classes. Having evolved from dance forms, the movements used in these classes should be screened to meet the safety and effectiveness parameters of group exercise. For example, many of the disjointed, ballistic movements of funk-style dance should be modified for group fitness safety. Additionally, class components should fulfill specific fitness objectives so that the programs are not simply dance classes. For example, aerobic components should be continuous and sustain appropriate intensities. Themed classes, such as holiday themes, can also provide stylistic variations that add fun and festivity to programming. Boot camp classes offering military-style training and mind-body low-impact classes are other popular programming variations. A good aerobics class is fun and creative, while maintaining safety and efficacy.

Glossary

Add-on – A choreographic building technique in which one movement is taught before the next movement is added. This can be repeated to teach longer sequences of movement.

Axial movement – Movement that occurs above a stationary base where the central axis of the body holds a fixed spatial point.

Beats – Regular pulsations that have an even rhythm and occur in a continuous pattern of strong and weak pulsations.

Choreography – The planning and composition of structural movement.

Combinations – Two or more movement patterns combined and repeated in sequence several times in a row.

Continuous format – A method of aerobic training in which intensity is gradually increased until target hearts rates are achieved and then sustained for the duration of the aerobic component of class.

Directional cues – Visual or verbal cues that tell participants in which direction to move.

Downbeat – The regular strong pulsation in music occurring in a continuous pattern at an even rhythm.

Duple meter – Groupings of two beats, alternating stressed and unstressed pulses or beats.

Elements of variation – The ways in which base moves can be altered. Examples of elements of variation are lever, planar, directional, rhythmic, and intensity.

Footwork cues – Visual or verbal cues that tell participants which foot to move.

Freestyle method – Choreographic technique in which the cardiovascular segment of a class uses movements randomly chosen by the instructor.

Gallop – A movement in which the heel leads the step forward followed by a quick close of the other foot to it. As the weight shifts onto the second foot, the knee of the first leg is raised.

Gesturing leg – The non–weightbearing leg in any movement.

Hop – A step in which the body weight is propelled off the ground from one foot with the landing occurring on the same foot.

Horizontal impact – Impact created by friction that makes the foot slide less easily across the floor.

Intermittent training (Interval training) – Exercising at high-intensity levels for brief periods (10 seconds to 5 minutes) with intervening rest or relief periods at a lower intensity to allow the heart rate to decline.

Jump – A step in which the body weight is propelled from one or both feet with the landing occurring on both feet.

Layering – A choreographic building technique in which options for changing intensity, complexity, and impact are super-imposed on established movements.

Linear progression – Consists of one movement that transitions into another without cycling sequences.

Locomotor movement – Movement in which the central axis of the body changes its location as it travels through space.

Meter – The organization of beats into groups with the strongest beat occurring on count one.

Numerical cues – Visual or verbal cues instructors use to count the rhythm of the exercise, such as "1 and 2, 3, 4."

Phrase – Composed of at least two measures of music.

Repetition reduction – A teaching strategy involving reducing the number of repetitions that make up a movement sequence.

Rhythm – A regular pattern of movement or sound that can be felt, heard, or seen.

Rhythmic cues – Visual or verbal cues that indicate the correct rhythm of an exercise or step pattern, such as slow (2 counts) or quick (1 count).

Rhythmic variation – A variation that alters a movement's rhythm to create more or less movement per unit of time. An example is performing movements at half-tempo to allow participants to learn complex movements.

Run – A step in which there is a momentary loss of contact with the ground as the weight shifts from foot to foot.

Skip – A movement in which a step and a hop are performed sequentially on the same foot as the mover alternates feet.

Slide – A movement in which the mover steps sideways then draws the other foot up to the first with a quick transfer of weight.

Step cues – Visual or verbal cues that refer to the name of the step in an aerobics routine, such as "step, ball-change."

Structured method – Choreographic technique in which the cardiovascular segment uses formally arranged step patterns repeated in a predetermined order.

Syncopation – A rhythmic device that temporarily shifts the normal pattern of stressed to unstressed beats or parts of beats.

Tempo – The rate of speed of music, usually expressed in beats per minute.

Transitions – Connections between individual movements and blocks of movements.

Triple meter – Groupings of three beats with emphasis on the first beat.

Upbeat – The regular, weak pulsation in music occurring in a continuous pattern at an even rhythm.

Vertical impact – Force exerted upward through the foot.

Visual previews – A type of visual cueing in which participants continue performing established movements while the instructor demonstrates a new movement.

Walk – A step in which weight is transferred from foot to foot with one foot always remaining in contact with the ground.

Working leg – The weightbearing leg in any movement.

Index

A

add-on, 25-26, 64
aerobic-circuit training, 62-63
aerobic component, 54-57
aerobic cool-down, 57-58
aerobic dance-exercise.
    see aerobics
Aerobic Dancing, Inc., 1, 13
aerobic music services, 12
Aerobic Q-signs, 30
aerobics
    benefits, 2-3
    gender bias, 1-2
    growth, 2
    three primary types, 2
Aerobics (Cooper), 1
African dance–based classes, 63
American College of
    Sports Medicine, 54
American Sign Language, 30
American Sports Data, 2
anaerobic intervals, 55-56
ankle weights, 29, 41
anterior shoulder stretch, 59, 61
arm movements
    adding, 41
    and intensity, 40
    overhead, 40-41
arthritis, 38
attitude towards time, 21
audible cues, 36
axial movements, 17, 18, 64

B

balance, biomechanical,
    3-4, 23, 51
ball-changes, 46
ballet, 63
ballistic movements, 34, 63
bar, of music, 9
basic movement variations, 14-15
beat, moving to the, 6-7
beats, 7, 64
beats per minute (bpm), 7
bench stepping, 40
beta blockers, 37
bilateral patterning, 45
biomechanical balance,
    3-4, 23, 51
biomechanics, knowledge of,
    34, 60
blood pooling, 57, 58
body, 19
    position of in space, 22-23
body fat, 38
body language corrections, 32
body orientation cues, 33
boot camp classes, 63
breath awareness, 58

C

cardiovascular fitness, 38, 54
center of gravity, raising and
    lowering, 42-43, 48

L

Laban, R., 21
Latin dance–based classes, 63
layering, 26, 44, 46, 65
lead leg reverses, 23-24
lever element of variation, 19, 20
lever length modifications, 41
lifting, 41
linear progressions, 16, 51, 65
locomotor movements, 17-18, 65
low back stretch, 59, 61
low-impact aerobics, 2, 47-48
lumbar lordosis, 38
lumbar spinal forward flexion, 35
lunge stretch, 60
lunges, 24

M

mats, 28
maximal heart rate (MHR), 54
measure, of music, 9
medical conditions, 37-38
meter, musical, 9-10, 65
Mettler, B., 12
mind-body low-impact classes, 63
mirror image, transitioning
     from or to, 24
mirrors, 28, 36
Missett, Judi Sheppard, 1, 13
mixed-impact aerobics, 2
moderate-impact aerobics, 48
modern dance–based classes, 63
modifications
     for complexity, 44-46
     cueing, 32
     for impact, 46-49
     for intensity, 39-44
     lever length, 41
     for medical conditions, 37-38
     review of, 27

monitoring, intensity,
     36, 37, 60-62
motivation, 38
motivational cue, 32
movement, structuring, 15-16
movement classification, 17-22
movement patterning, 13-17
moving to the beat, 6-7
multi-level classes, 44, 56
muscle-conditioning intervals,
     56-57
muscle imbalances, 38
muscular-endurance training, 58
music
     counting, 8
     election of appropriate, 12
     interpretation, 6-12
     levels, 29, 36
     licensing, 29
     meter, 9
     music beats, 6-7
     musicians' counts, 8
     phrases, 10-11
     tempo, 7-9, 53

N

neutral pelvis, stabilizing,
     35, 36, 37
non-weightbearing leg.
     see gesturing leg
numerical cues, 31, 32, 65

O

Occupational Safety and Health
     Administration (OSHA), 29
Oliva, G. A., 30
Otto, R., 44
overuse injuries, 34

P

pain, 27
pelvic tilts, 51, 52
pelvis, neutral, stabilizing, 35, 36, 37
personal limitations, 37-39
phrase, musical, 10-11, 65
planar, 19, 20
platform, instructor, 28, 36
pliés, 51
PNF stretching, 59
position of body in space, 22-23
pre-exercise screening, 34
pregnancy, 38
pre-performance stretching, 54
programming
    components, 50-60
    intensity monitoring, 36, 37, 60-62
    variations, 62-63
progression, rate of, 34, 53
propulsions, 23, 43, 48
pulse monitoring, 27, 61
push releases, 52-53
pyramid building, 24-25

R

raised platform, 36
range of motion, 34
range of movements, and intensity, 42, 43
rate of progression, 34, 53
rating of perceived exertion (RPE), 37, 61-62
    chart, 28
recovery intervals, 55-56
regular tempo, 11
rehearsal, 51, 53
repetition reduction, 24-25, 46, 65
resistance apparatus, 28
rhythm, 11-12, 65

rhythmic cues, 31, 32, 65
rhythmic element of variation, 19, 21, 25, 66
rhythmic patterns, of movement and music, 6, 11
Rizzo, T. H., 28
room temperature, 35
run, 17, 66

S

scoots, 23
secondary rhythms, 11
set, 57
shin splints, 48
shoes. *see* footwear
shoulder rolls, 51, 52
skip, 18, 66
slide, 18, 66
social interaction, 2
soleus stretch, 59
Sorensen, Jacki, 1, 13
sound system, 28
space, 19, 29, 35
    position of body in, 22-23
spatial cues, 33-34
spatial element of variation, 19-21
sports-conditioning programs, 62
squats, 23
stability, 35
stability balls, 28
standing pelvic tilts, 51
static stretching, 54, 59
steady-state training, 55, 61
step aerobics, 2
step cues, 31, 66
step-touch, 18
stillness, 58
strength training, 58
stress reduction, 58
stretching, 58-60, 61, 62

References and Suggested Reading

American Sports Data, Inc. (1996). Hartsdale, New York.

Clippinger, K. (1993). *Aerobics Instructor Manual.* San Diego, Calif.: American Council on Exercise, 206.

Cohen, B.B. (1993). *Sensing, Feeling and Action.* Northampton, Mass.: Contact Editions, 101.

Copeland, C. (1987). *Moves, the Foolproof Formula for Creative Choreography.* Los Angeles: CompuThink, Inc., 29–44.

Ellison, D. (1996). *Flexible Strength.* Canton, Mass.: Reebok University Press, 14.

Francis, L. (1993). *Aerobics Instructor Manual.* San Diego, Calif.: American Council on Exercise, 260.

Francis, P. & Francis, L. (1988). Weighty Issues, *IDEA Today*, 6, 8, 47–49.

Francis, P. & Francis, L. (1989). High- and low-impact aerobics, *IDEA Today*, 7, 7, 56–63.

Francis, P. & Francis, L. (1989). Moderate Impact Aerobics, *IDEA Today*, 7, 8, 27–29.

Francis, P. & Francis, L. (1992). Effects of choreography, step height, fatigue, and gender on metabolic cost of step training, *Medicine & Science in Sports & Exercise*, abstract 69, Supplement 24, 5.

Garrick, J., Gillien, D., & Whiteside, P. (1986). Epidemiology of Aerobic Dance Injuries, *American Journal of Sports Medicine*, Jan/Feb, 14, 1.

Gavin, J. (1997). Something in the Way You Move. *IDEA Today,* 15, 6, 25–27.

Griffith, B.R. (1982). *Dance for Fitness.* Minneapolis, Minn.: Burgess Publishing Co.

Guest, A.H. (1995). *Your Move, A New Approach to the Study of Movement and Dance.* Gordon and Breach Publishers. 279–285.

Kagan, E. & Morse, M. (1988). The Body Electronic: Aerobic Exercise on Video. *The Drama Review,* 32, 4, 166.

Kapandji, I.A. (1974). *The Physiology of the Joints.* New York: Churchill Livingstone, 150.

Laban, R. (1974). *The Mastery of Movement.* Boston: Plays, Inc. 75–89.

Laban, R. (1976). *The Language of Movement.* Boston: Plays, Inc. 18–26.

Lauffenburger, S.K. (1986). Aiding Pelvic Alignment, *Dance Exercise Today,* 2, 6, 34–35.

Mettler, B. (1979). *Materials of Dance as a Creative Art Activity.* Tuscon, Ariz.: Mettler Studios, 168, 191, 76.

Nottingham, S. (1998). Group Exercise Becomes of Age, *Fitness Management,* 14, 6, 39.

Oliva, G.A. (1988). *Visual Cues for Exercise Classes.* Washington, D.C.: Gallaudet University.

Otto, R., Yoke, M., Wygand, R., & Kamimokai, C. (1988). The Metabolic Cost of Two Differing Low Impact Aerobic Dance Exercise Modes, *Medicine & Science in Sports & Exercise,* 20–2 (abstract), 525.

Pollack, M. & Wilmore, J. (1990). *Exercise in Health and Disease.* Philadelphia, Penn.: W.B.Saunders.

Rizzo, T.H. (1999). Choosing Athletic Shoes, *IDEA Health and Fitness Source,* 17, 5, 28–39.

Simmons, R. (1998). The Critical Loop in Quality Instruction, *IDEA Fitness Edge,* 1, 5, 4–6.

Tech, K. (1994). *Ear Training for the Body.* Pennington, N.J.: Princeton Book Company, 44.

Webb, T. (1989). Aerobic Q-Signs. *IDEA Today*, 10, 30–31.

NOTES

NOTES

NOTES

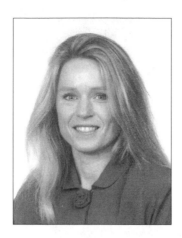

Kathryn Bricker, B.S., C.M.A., is a certified Laban movement analyst, American Council on Exercise continuing education provider, and ACE Gold-certified Group Fitness Instructor. She is a former chairperson of ACE's group fitness certification committee and has served on ACE's item writing and role delineation committees. Bricker has been instructing group fitness full-time since 1979.